DOING IT!

One woman's guide to a healthier body and mind.

Nic Doward

Illustrated by Darryl Doward

Copyright © 2023 Darryl Doward

All rights reserved.

DLDowardart.com

@DLDowardart

Copyright © 2023 Nic Doward

All rights reserved.

ISBN: 9798857019580

nicdowardcoaching.com

DEDICATION

Darryl, Abi and Sophie – you have loved and supported me no matter what.

To anyone who struggles with obesity: I know your pain. I feel your frustration and want you to know that it is possible.

To everyone who runs, pushes a pram, jogs, walks or crawls and to anyone who wants to run, push a pram, jog, walk or crawl.

We are not alone x

CONTENTS

	Acknowledgements	Pg 7
1	Once upon a time…	Pg 13
2	If only there'd been signs	Pg 25
3	All in the mind	Pg 39
4	Eating with the enemy	Pg 57
5	Graft	Pg 76
6	If only it were that simple	Pg 90
7	Running up that hill	Pg 104
8	Food for thought	Pg 117
9	Run, Nic, Run!	Pg 124
10	Doing it!	Pg 137

ACKNOWLEDGMENTS

I am not a weight loss expert. I am not a fitness expert. I only know what is working for me. I have written this book because I had eaten myself to death's door and I am pulling myself back.

Two things helped me to pull myself back.

The first is knowing that I am not alone. I know this through the love and support of the following gorgeous people:

My family - immediate and extended. There aren't enough words other than I love you.

The marshals at Warrington Parkrun – they are the best of the rest of us and I thank them for being so wonderful from the bottom of my heart. They have saved my life. The Warrington Parkrun community – wonderfully, decent, kind and encouraging people. Every Saturday, they turn up, they do the thing and they lift each other doing it. They lift me. I often find myself smiling throughout my 5K - grimacing, sweating, swearing… but smiling. There is one gentleman, John, who tells me every time we pass - 'go on girl - you're doing it!' It gets me every time. I used to stand over by the tree, hiding, until one wonderful woman, Katie, came over one week to invite me to join the pack. I could write a thousand of these snippets of goodness like these - all of them have helped me to keep on 'doing it'. Infact, the Parkrun community worldwide is just tremendous. When I wrote my post on Facebook (you'll get to it), I was overwhelmed by the responses. It showed me that there are way more good people in the world than bad. Most people are trying. People actually want you to do well. I had been hiding from the world for so long and I really needed that affirmation of humanity.

Jo - my walking companion and my friend - when we get to the field, she finds her second wind and it powers both of us home. When she shouts 'come on Nic, breathe', I do it. I don't dare do otherwise. She is Mickey to my Rocky!

Bev, the best aqua instructor in the world bar none, is a real life example of what is possible. She's lost 11 stone and is now a full time fitness instructor. She motivates, she challenges and she supports - her set lists are also fabulous and I often find myself singing along like a deranged lunatic whilst punching the water.

I never thought of myself as a yoga person. I thought yoga was for super fit, super chill and very zen people - basically, not me. I was so very wrong. My sister in law

Beverley encouraged me to join her at a beginners slow flow class and the instructor Lauren is just brilliant. Her classes are beautiful. I know that's a weird word to describe a fitness class but it is the best word for them. She makes me feel capable and strong. She has shown me that time not thinking actually helps me to think, that discomfort can be growth and that being kind to yourself is most important of all.

Lastly, Animas Coaching, Lillian and our wonderful group - I have practised professional coaching for years but this year I threw myself into a Transformational Coaching qualification. As I have deepened my learning and practice, I have been able to apply this to my own life and began to understand my own thinking and behaviour much more clearly. I have had the benefit of being coached by the wonderful practitioners in my group - they have helped me to reflect and have given me the space to grow, the grace to own my failures and the strength to find a different way.

The second thing that helped to pull me back was knowing it was possible. My aqua instructor Bev is a real life example of what can be achieved. She has done it. She stands before our class and she does every step with us. I look at her and I see that it is possible. My biggest mindshift though came from Parkrun. No-one looked at me like I didn't belong. Quite the opposite. They treated me like it was normal for me to be there. Like I was normal... like I was just like them. I remember a woman running past me once and as she passed she said, 'I know - we all feel the pain. Keep going'. It was a moment of human connection - in a split second, she saw me, she understood me and she offered me comfort. It was momentary. Every Saturday, the Parkrun community does that over and over again. Moments of human kindness and connection being delivered by real life models of what can be. They have shown me, in all of their extraordinary 'normalness' that it is possible.

These two things have combined at a time when I needed them most. I still need them. I am still doing it. I will always be doing it. If I take my starting point as 31 stone / 434 lbs / 197 kg, I have lost over 8 and a half stone / 119lbs / 54 kg at this point. In actual fact, I know I was way above 31 stone because my weighing scales only measure up to 31 stone and it hadn't registered me for a long time. When I came home from France in August 2022, I stepped on the scales and I was overjoyed when it registered me at 30 stone 1lb. By my first Parkrun, I had tipped under 30 stone - who'd have thought seeing 29 stone on a scale would bring me such joy! At the time of publication, August 2023, nearly 1 year to my first PR and 1 year into doing it, I am nearly 8 and a half stone

(119 lbs / 54 kg) lighter. My next milestone is to get under 20 stone and become a teenager again!

Knowing how these two things have helped me, I wanted to reach out to those who are also struggling. One of my coaching colleagues, Nikki, shared a wonderful quote from Morgan Harper Nichols 'Tell the story of the mountain you climbed. Your words could become a page in someone else's survival guide.' I have not finished my mountain - I believe I am going to be climbing this one for the rest of my days. But it is my hope that this book will be the metaphorical and literal first pages of your story.

I want you to know that you are not alone. You will have people in your life who love you and want the best for you. It is hard to see that sometimes. At the very least, reading this, you will know that wherever you are, I am right here and I am still doing it. Same as you. We are not alone. And we both know that it is possible. Together we have the will and together we will find the way. How do I know? Because we will not stop - we are doing it!

Chapter 1

Once upon a time…

In October 2022, I posted something on the Warrington Parkrun facebook page. I did it because I'd been walking Parkrun since August 2022 and, in those 2 short months, it was already changing my life. No exaggeration. I knew what it was doing for me and I hoped that sharing my story might help someone else who felt 'the fear.' So I sat down to write:

On 19th August 2022, I gathered all of my courage and registered for parkrun. At just under 190 kilograms (30 stone), the three 'M's were a daily battle; morbid obesity, mobility and mortality. I was literally at the point of 'do or die'.

My husband, Darryl, and daughter, Sophie are Parkrunners. They'd told me so many times that it was for everyone: all ages, all sizes, all abilities. 'Sure!' I thought, 'but not my size, not my ability.' I was too embarrassed to even go to watch. Darryl reassured me that no one would judge.

So on 20th August, I turned up and did my first parkrun, well parkwalk! My husband was right (first time for everything!), I did not feel judged. In fact, I can honestly say that the parkrun community is one of the most inclusive, welcoming and encouraging communities I've ever experienced.
First of all, I am never last. There is always a tail walker who has that honour. Tracey was the tail walker on my very first parkwalk. She was patient, kind, supportive and so encouraging. Since then I've walked with Rob, Kim, Richard, Christina - all have been incredibly supportive.

My first Parkwalk took me an hour and 26 minutes. Not one volunteer made me feel guilty for keeping them out at their posts. They were all genuinely encouraging and supportive. I cried quite a few times during that one. The first tears were exhaustion and fear of not being able to finish, the last ones, at the finish line, were tears of joy because I had actually done it. The volunteers had all stayed, even though the person in front of me finished 30 minutes before. They cheered for me with the same enthusiasm and respect as they do for the front runners! I do not have enough words to express how much I appreciate each and every one of them.
I didn't expect everyone else to be just as supportive, but they were. I cannot tell you how many times I've felt, 'I can't take another step,' and then a fellow Parkrunner/walker will give me a nod, a thumbs up, a, 'well done,' or, 'keep going,' and it fills me with a determination to walk on. On my third time, by

about the 4k mark, I literally thought I cannot take another step. A woman appeared from nowhere, walked alongside me, talked to me about how to breathe. She walked me to the finish line and then disappeared. To this day, I don't know who she was. She wasn't a volunteer, she'd just done the run herself! I even feared I'd imagined her but my Sophie reassured me that she was real.

I now look forward to Saturday mornings. Darryl, Sophie and I all go. They finish in their own time and then walk back to meet me. Sophie walks alongside me and paces me to get over the finish line. I am just back from my seventh event and I completed the course in one hour and four minutes. I am determined to get under the hour.

Richard, the tail walker, with the gift of holding a conversation when my contributions are single words and grunts, mentioned to me today that parkrun has launched a parkwalk initiative to let people know that you are just as welcome to join in whether you wish to run or walk or do a bit of both. As a walker, I wanted to share my story. If I can do it, anyone can! Having completed seven parkwalks, I'm by no means a seasoned athlete, but I'm heading in the right direction and even more importantly, I now actually believe I can do this. I look forward to my Saturday mornings. Completing the 5k is still hard but getting to the finish line is the best feeling ever. I notice my mood has improved, my energy levels are so much higher and those three 'M's aren't as much of a battle anymore. I am 'doing' and I love it.

So if you have the fear I had, put it to one side. Register. Turn up. Do your best. I guarantee you – it's so much more than just a walk in the park!

I happened to be on the way to Ireland to visit family the day I posted that. Whilst in the car on the way to Holyhead, I started to get comments on my post. I began to reply to the comments to thank people for their support but soon found that they were coming in quicker than I could respond. Infact, the response to the post was so huge that Facebook actually blocked me because I think they thought I was a bot!

When the 'likes' reached into the thousands and the comments just kept coming, I realised something that broke and fixed my heart in one fell swoop: I was not alone. I was not the only one struggling with my weight. I was not the only one who was scared to try something new. But I was also not the only one who was trying to do something about it. I had stumbled into a community of positive, kind and affirming people who made me feel like anything is possible. I got messages from my fellow Warrington Parkrunners - the ones who had been encouraging me from day one. I even got messages from across the globe! Every message gave me the confidence

and self belief that one day I would achieve the impossible: complete the 5K in under 1 hour!
It seems that registering for Parkrun on the 19th August set off a domino effect which was a catalyst for something so much more. That simple act was a commitment to making a change. Since then, I have been doing Parkrun/walk every week - rain, hail or shine. As I reflect upon my journey across this year, I realise that committing to doing that one thing, and the domino effect thereafter, has added up to a whole lot of change for me. I realise that up to that point, the enormity of what I had to do was just too much to face. I couldn't see myself being able to change everything so I didn't change anything. The night I registered for Parkrun, I did one thing. The next day, I walked. I got through those very hard and scary days with one focus - get a little bit faster.

That singular focus flipped my thinking. I was no longer overwhelmed by the enormity of the task ahead of me - all I had to do was to walk a little bit faster than the week before. All of a sudden it was achievable.

This gave me the time, space and perspective to find my ultimate goal - to be fit and healthy in body and mind. I stopped obsessing about my weight and what I needed to deprive myself of and instead I started focusing on what I needed **to do**! I motivated myself by thinking about what it would feel like to achieve my goal - I would feel healthy, fit, capable, free, strong. I thought about what that would look like – yes, I would have a smaller body but it was more than that. I would have muscles! I would be able to buy clothes in 'normal' shops at 'normal' prices. I wouldn't have to wear tent t-shirts emblazoned with butterflies and random words anymore. I would be able to move. I would be able to walk up my stairs without taking breaks. I would be able to run up my stairs! If I achieved this, I would have a chance to see my children graduate, get jobs, have children ….I would live. I know that sounds dramatic but this is what it means to me.

And all I had to do to achieve all of that is to try to walk a little bit faster than I did the week before! I was, and still am, giddy with the possibilities. I'd spent my life looking for the light at the end of the tunnel and I'd just found out that I was holding the light. The light was right here in my hand and had been all along!

This is why I am writing this. If you have ever found yourself stuck in the cycle of dieting and self sabotaging, you will understand what I'm sharing. I'm inviting you to embark on your own journey as you read through this book with me. At the end of each chapter, I'm going to ask you the questions I asked myself and I want you to be truly honest with yourself. I am leaving you space to jot down a few notes - committing something to paper somehow multiplies its potency!

By the way, I am not at the end of my journey. I have lost 8 and a half stone in the past 11 months and my life is totally different to what it was. I am changed because my thinking has changed. I continue to work at it. We are in this together.

Your turn:

What is it that you want to achieve?

How will you know you have achieved your goal? How will you measure success?

What does success in this goal **look** like? Try to be as detailed as possible.

What does success in this goal **feel** like? Again, get right into the detail.

What difference would it make in your life if you achieved this?

What would happen if you didn't achieve your goal?

_____
_____
_____
_____
_____
_____
_____
_____
_____
_____
_____
_____
_____
_____
_____
_____
_____
_____

On a scale of 1-10, how important is it to you that you achieve this?

       1 2 3 4 5 6 7 8 9 10

Not important   Very Important

Well then, let's do it!

Chapter 2

If only there'd been signs

I don't actually know what my top weight was. I know I had reached over 31 stone / 434 lbs / 197 kg because my scales had a maximum capacity of 31 stone, but it had been a long time since they had even registered my weight. By July 2022, I was in a bad way. I was in size 36 clothes. My blood pressure was through the roof, as was my cholesterol, I was pre-diabetic ready to tip into full blown diabetes and my quality of life was at an all time low. I felt like my heart was going to burst out of my chest several times a day. I said in the FB post that I felt that I was at the point of 'do or die' and I was not exaggerating. I was very scared.

The question that haunts me is 'how did I get to that point?' I mean getting to a weight of over 31 stone does not happen overnight and I can't quite believe that I let it get so bad.

If only there'd been signs along the way that could have shown me where I was headed, maybe I could have avoided becoming so unhealthy.

Except there was.

Like the time I went to see the stage play of the musical Dirty Dancing with friends. It was a brilliant production and I thoroughly enjoyed it - except for the fact that at some point during the performance, the base of the seat I was sitting on gave way under my weight. It was one of those seats that flipped up and down and it simply collapsed under me. I was mortified - there was no way I was going to stand up in the middle of the show and report that I had broken it.

Luckily, the seat was so narrow that I was wedged right in there so while gravity was working against me, the overspill of my girth was applying an immovable force to stop me slipping down. I girded my arms and fixed my legs to maintain my seated pose, wedged into that seat, right till the end of the show. When I finally stood, my legs were so numb I could barely move. I joked with my friends that Johnny had made my knees go weak. I didn't dare tell them the truth. That really should have been a sign.

While no one puts Baby in a corner, life very often put me in seats that were just not built for the bigger bottom! I 'got away' with the incident above but I was not so lucky whilst on holiday in France with the family in 2022. We had passed a lovely restaurant a number of times and, one evening, we decided to treat ourselves and went inside. We were shown to our table on the patio which could not have been more picturesque. Only problem was that the chairs were aluminium garden chairs with rigid arm rests. I knew the minute I sat down that I was in trouble. The chairs were so narrow that it was only the sheer force of my weight which forced me down into it that allowed me to sit in the chair at all. I could feel those steel bars digging into the sides of my legs and my hips for the duration of the meal. I didn't want to ruin the experience for my children and my husband so I didn't tell them how much pain I was in. However, when we finished our mains, I finally admitted that the chair was hurting 'a little.' I said that I would go to the bathroom and then wait for them outside. The chair had different plans for me. I attempted to stand only to find that the chair was rising with me. I sat back down. I tried one more time but the same thing happened. The bum was well and truly stuck! The problem was that my upper body had spilled over the armrests which meant that I could not access them to lever myself out of the chair. I leaned forward and whispered to my family that I was stuck. 'What do you mean, 'stuck'?' Darryl asked. I explained that I was wedged into the chair and that when I stood up, the chair was rising up with me. As I said it out loud, the ridiculousness of the situation hit me and I began to giggle. The giggle turned to a laugh and the laugh turned into uncontrollable cackles. Tears were running down my face - to this day I don't quite know if it was the laughter or the embarrassment that triggered them. In the end, Darryl, the husband, stood behind me and pretended to be casually leaning on the back of my chair to hold it down as I stood and unwedged myself. We like to pretend that this farce was so smooth that one noticed but we all know that there wasn't a person in that restaurant who didn't know what was going on. The bruises on the sides of my legs were deep and painful but nothing hurts as much as the memory.

Holidays actually gave me so many signs but I shall select just one more holiday riddled with signs that I just couldn't/wouldn't see. Summer holidays again, this time it was during that 'eat out to help out' covid madness in 2020. We decided to go to Newcastle for a week and use it as a base to see Northumberland. Great plan - except my mobility was zero. I'd had to isolate during covid due to being morbidly obese and, by the time of this holiday, I couldn't walk for any length of time. In fact, just standing was exhausting. When we went out as a family, my mobility seriously limited what we could do and so, more and more, I just opted out till I had almost become a recluse. My mental health was not good and, in truth, I was very unwell in body and mind.

Nonetheless, we needed a holiday as a family and I decided that I was getting back out there. I was going to go out with the family and face the world. Except, I literally couldn't walk. I was actually using a walking stick for everyday use as my hips and knees would often just give way. So, I decided I would look into getting wheelchairs whilst out and about. Not as simple as I first thought though. Example: we had a day out at Alnwick Castle - absolutely fabulous and well worth the visit. Sophie was an avid Harry Potter fan so to visit the OG Hogwarts was a real treat. Ahead of time, I had booked myself an electric mobility scooter from the castle mobility centre - brilliant service by the way. The woman who handed over the scooter could not have been nicer - she was so gentle and generous with her time and did not make me feel judged at all. And the scooter meant that I was able to tour the grounds with the family - sure, I crashed into walls and nearly ran over a few toes - those things can move - but I soon got the hang of it. I was actually very proud of how I manoeuvred it when we went into a cafe for a bit of lunch. By that point, I was like an expert forklift driver on that thing. Unfortunately, just as we got settled, the fire alarm went off and the whole castle had to be evacuated. I will never forget the sound of the beeping scooter as I tried to reverse it out of the cafe amid the crowds of people desperately trying to evacuate. Another fit of giggles resulted in me being unable to even see what I was doing - which was lucky because the carnage of knocked over tables and chairs was not pretty. If there had been an actual fire, I would've resigned myself to just going up in smoke. Luckily, it was a false alarm.

Same holiday, using a different wheelchair, we had beeping of another variety to contend with. We went to the mobility centre of a shopping mall so that we could do a little bit of retail therapy. They did not have an electric scooter for my weight - but they did root around to find a push wheelchair that could accommodate me. Those things are not easy to move - especially with me in it. I couldn't self propel so Darryl stepped up to push me. I tried to help a little but it was mostly down to him to get me moving. As we 'glided' through the shopping mall, Darryl did his very best, despite the dips and slopes leading from one section to the other. All of a sudden, his Garmin watch starts beeping - turns out that the watch had detected that his heart was beating at an abnormally fast rate: pushing me was taking it out of him. When I heard this, I jumped up out of the chair and told him to sit in it. He refused, insisting that he was ok. I wouldn't hear of it and so began a heated argument about who should sit in the chair. Eventually, the youngest one, Sophie, jumped in the chair so that at least someone was in it. You would think that would have been enough to make me realise that enough is enough and I had to make a change.

It was not.

I am ashamed to say that it wasn't till July 2022 that I really realised how serious my situation was. I finally made the decision that my life had to be different or I would not survive.

I realise now that it didn't matter how many 'signs' that were thrown at me: until I was ready to open my eyes, to accept my reality and to accept that only I could fix it, I was never going to get better.

When I registered for the Parkrun, I was accepting responsibility for my condition and I was making a decision to live life differently. I was pushing myself way out of my comfort zone and I was making myself accountable. It was a metaphorical moment of pulling the plaster off.
I knew what I wanted - to be fit and healthy in body

and mind.

And, in fairness to me, in July 2022, I was trying. I wanted that summer holiday to be different so I had stopped eating chocolate which was my drug of choice. I was walking around the block at night time - 600 metres and it took about 30 minutes as I had to have so many rest breaks. Whilst on holiday in August, I made a point to swim every day. (Another sign - we went to the pool early on our first day, no one was there so in I get, via the very steep steps. Darryl helped me so all was good. Then another family arrived. And another and so on... I was done swimming but I couldn't get out of the pool. I was too embarrassed to ask Darryl to help me out in front of the other families and I couldn't hoosh myself up the steps. I ended up staying in that pool for 4 HOURS - until everyone had left and Darryl could help me out. I have Irish skin and I burn at the best of times. I was like a broiled lobster!)

During that holiday, my daughters Sophie and Abi would walk with me in the evening, counting out my steps and holding me up when my legs gave way. They would point out little markers and encourage me to make it to the next one and the one after the next night. I did not allow myself to opt out of family activities like I had done so many times before. I made myself go. I was in pain for that whole holiday but I did not stay home alone for a single activity. When we went out, the girls walked slowly on either side of me, pretending to be linking my arms. They were really helping me to walk. I feared, I think we all did, that it would be my last holiday. I had missed out on so much with them and I wanted the girls, and Darryl, to have some nice memories. I wanted to have some nice memories.

But a funny thing happened - the more I walked, the more I could walk. One day, just before we came home, I managed 5,000 steps in a day. Now this was a huge achievement for me coming from the 700 steps max I was managing before the holiday.

What's more, I didn't want the holiday where I got stuck in a chair AND a pool to be the last family holiday we had together. One day we went to an adventure park -I couldn't believe it when I read that the weight limit for the bungee jump was 217 KG (34 stone). I had always wanted to do a bungee jump and I was high on having done 3,000 steps the day before so I felt like anything was possible! I couldn't of course - the 34 stone limit was for a tandem jump. They didn't have a harness big enough to fit me. Trying to piece together that question in my pigeon french to ask the attendant was not a highlight of the holiday:

Excuse-moi,c'est ok pour moi de faire ça parce que je suis très gros?' Excuse me - is it ok for me to do this because I am very fat?

'Non'

But the important thing is that I wanted to do it. I wanted to live. I knew that I needed to do something.

So when I got home, I registered for Parkrun. I had not walked 5K before I did my first one. I did not know if I would be able to finish.

I only knew that I had to take the first step.

Your turn:

So now - what is the first step in your journey? What is the one thing you are going to do to set your dominoes in motion?

Why have you chosen to do this?

When / where are you going to do it?

Will you do it on your own or with someone else?

What could stop you from achieving this?

If you've identified a blocker, how can you get around it?

Look at what you have written. You have your first step: what, where, when, with whom, what, if anything could stop you AND how to get around that.

Well done!

Now go do it.

Chapter 3

All in the mind

Now I have spent my whole life believing that I am fat. Even more than that, I believed that being a fat woman was about as bad a thing as I could be. I was filled with shame.

Looking back at photographs, I see that the truth is that I actually wasn't always fat. I think I ate myself into being the vision I had of me in my mind's eye since childhood. I wasn't fat but believing I was had paved the way for me to become so.

When I say I wasn't fat, what I mean is that I was 'normal'. I wasn't 'thin' but neither was I overweight. The era of body positivity had not yet dawned and being beautiful meant being rake thin. I was not that. That made me feel self conscious and so I comforted myself - with food. And so began a cycle of torment that would last right up to ...well August 2022!

This wasn't a cycle of my own creation now - it is tried and tested across the world. You may even recognise it yourself.

What's more, the world constantly and consistently reinforced it.

For example, during a performance review at work many years ago, my line manager congratulated me on a very successful year. I had achieved all of my objectives and had surpassed my targets. Well done me! Then it came to objective setting for the forthcoming year and my boss told me that he knew that whatever I set my mind to in work, I would achieve it. My work ethic was second to none and he would agree to whatever objectives I wanted to set. I think he just wanted me to fill in the paperwork. BUT he had one thing he would like me to think about. I should lose weight. If I wanted people to take me seriously, I needed to lose weight because no-one would see how good I was, at the size I was.

I was a size 18.

I thanked him for the review and walked out of that office burning with shame. If it happened now, I would like to think that I'd give him a piece of my mind (goodness knows he needed it with having so very little of his own to think with). But back then, it was par for the course. I was 'fat'. People would assume I was lazy. I should lose weight. That was my professional development for that year!

This has been a battle for me my whole life. I have tried everything at one time or another: weight loss tablets - prescribed and dodgy internet ones - Weight Watchers, Slimming World, Slimfast, Atkins, Cabbage soup, Cambridge… they all work, when you work them (except the dodgy internet tablets - codswallop!).

For me, the problem has really always been in my head. I would start well, lose a lot of weight and feel great. Then my body would realise that something was going on and the weight loss would slow down. I would get frustrated. Frustration would turn to despair and despair would turn to self loathing …… leading to comfort eating and the slippery slope where I would put it all back on. And more.

I even got a gastric band fit 15 years ago! It's still in! That's right - I blew up to over 31 stone with a gastric band. That was probably one of the worst decisions I have ever made. Actually scratch that - it served a purpose.

As I mentioned, I've always been big but I became seriously overweight in my 30s. I had my first daughter Abi when I was 29 - we got pregnant on honeymoon and, whilst it was sooner than we expected, we were both delighted.

Unfortunately, when I was 3 months pregnant my mother had a fatal stroke. It was out of the blue and shocked us all.

We found out I was pregnant in Singapore airport on the way back from our honeymoon – I only bought the pregnancy test because we had time to kill between flights. We decided there and then not to tell anyone till the 12 week scan. When we got home, I called my ma to tell her we were back safe and sound … and the first thing that I blurted out was 'I'm pregnant'. She was so excited for us. I am the youngest of 10 children and my ma was a baby whisperer. When my sisters had had their children, my ma had always been there in those early days to help, hold and comfort - she also helped with the baby! It was a rite of passage that I was so looking forward to.

I had had my 12 week scan just before the half term holiday – perfect timing as I was going back to Ireland for the holiday and I couldn't wait to show everyone the scan picture. Darryl and I lived in England so I hadn't seen my family since the day after our wedding in August. It was a brilliant wedding and we both had a ball but it had been hectic and then we had flown off on honeymoon the very next day. I couldn't wait to talk about the wedding, the honeymoon, being pregnant…and more than anything, I just wanted a hug from my ma.

I got the call just days before I was due to travel. My ma had collapsed with a major stroke and was in a very serious condition. I booked the first available flight. I remember holding my purse with my scan picture in it just praying that she would come around and I would be able to show it to her. It was almost like a talisman - she'd have to come round to see the scan! She didn't come round. The doctors told us that the brain damage was irrevocable and we made the tough decision to turn off her life support. She slipped away very peacefully surrounded by those that loved her.

I remember crying in the hospital and someone said to me that my ma would want me to think of the baby now. If I was upset, the baby would be upset and that wouldn't be good for them. They meant well and it did help to focus on the baby. But after that, whenever I felt sad or missed my ma, I did not let myself feel it. I squished it up and pushed it down so hard that it just compacted inside me. I did not let myself grieve.

Then I had Abi. I was totally unprepared for the torrent of emotions that engulfs you when you have a child. I expected the love but the power of it was overwhelming. I didn't fully expect the fear. People talk about the fear but you don't actually get it till it is right on top of you. The responsibility of it was huge – I was supposed to be a mammy and all I wanted was my mammy. I did not feel up to the job at all. And to top it all off, the tiredness just seemed to deepen with each day. As these emotions swirled in my brain, my grief saw its chance and it broke free. I was not a well woman.

I turned to food for comfort. Chocolate in particular but in truth it didn't matter what it was - I just ate and ate and ate ... but nothing could fill the hole inside of me.

I got up to 24 stone and that was the heaviest I'd been up to that point. I was desperate to lose the weight. I had a 2 year old child who was very active and I was struggling to keep up with her. I also wanted another child but our first pregnancy was high risk because I was 16 stone -I knew that going into another pregnancy 8 stone heavier was too risky.

So I decided to get a gastric band. In my head, it made sense - the band would limit how much I could eat. If I couldn't over eat, then I would lose weight. Presto skinny me, and another baby to boot. It sounded too good to be true - I later found out that it was.

I lost a huge chunk of the weight that time before the surgery. They have you go on a very strict diet before the surgery to shrink your liver. The weight flew off. After the surgery, you have to go on a liquid diet while you heal - shakes or soups for breakfast, lunch, dinner and tea! It worked. I lost weight, got to 18 stone and got pregnant! So it served a purpose.

I had talked with the clinic about why I wanted the band before I got it and they had said that it was perfectly safe over pregnancy. The band can be adjusted according to how tight you want it. If it is letting too much food pass through it, you can have saline injected into it to increase its 'grip'. If it is not letting enough food through, you can have saline removed from the band and it will loosen the 'grip'.

By the time I got pregnant with Sophie, I was actually eating very little. The strict diet, soups and shakes all diminish your appetite. However, once I found out I was pregnant, I knew I had to eat healthily. I tried but food would get 'stuck'. Getting 'stuck' means the food will not pass through the band, gets stuck in your oesophagus and it causes excruciating pain. The only way to stop the pain is to regurgitate it back up. Nice. Sometimes it was fine, sometimes I would have one bite and the food would get stuck and I would have to run to the bathroom to bring it back up.

I was worried about the baby getting the nutrients she needed. I went back to the clinic and asked them to remove the saline - which they did. The problem continued. The annoying thing is that if I ate anything oily or with cream, it just slipped through. However, when I tried to eat salad or crunchy vegetables for example, it would get stuck and I would have to run to the toilet to vomit. It seemed that the healthier the food, the bigger the risk of me being unable to eat it: steamed breast of chicken? Not a chance. Rocket salad? No way? Sticky toffee pudding and custard? No problem! Many meals have been ruined because I just can't eat the food in front of me. It has taken a long time to work out how to live with this thing and it still impacts on how I eat to this day.

I think back to the decision to have major surgery to lose weight and I can't quite believe I let myself do it. Of course, I know why I did it. Because I wanted Sophie.

That's a lie.

It was because I wanted a quick fix.

This is what I meant by looking for the light at the end of the tunnel - I was forever looking for a way to 'solve' me. I really thought something or someone else would be able to do it. Perhaps I had so little faith in myself that I just didn't think I could. I thought someone else, much more clever and capable than me, had the answer.

So whenever I embarked on a new diet or fad, I was doing someone else's plan. They all worked for a while but because they were not mine, I couldn't keep it up. They all involved me giving up something or depriving myself. I was on an endless cycle of punishing myself to lose weight, getting to a place bereft of joy and with very little reward …. leading me to finding comfort in food… The cycle was perpetual. My relationship with food has always been complex - it was my best friend and my worst enemy. It made me giddy with joy and riddled with self-loathing. I was addicted.

Extreme? Yes. True? Also yes. Problem was, I was surrounded by my drug. I had easy access to it every day. Indeed, people encouraged me to indulge – have a cake, have a biscuit, you deserve a treat. You'd never force an alcoholic to have a drink but I was often cajoled into having a desert. Don't get me wrong – I didn't need much cajoling. I have sabotaged myself more than anyone else has ever sabotaged me.

I had little routines that I thought were so clever when I wanted to hide what I was eating. For example, I have pretended to be on the phone with an imaginary friend when going through the drive through to pretend that I'm not buying 2 meals just for me. I have had different routes to work to pass different shops so that each shop doesn't know that the amount of chocolate I am buying is just for the car ride home and not the kids party/ cinema trip / family film night I was babbling on about. I mean, who were those little charades for?

For me.

My head liked to think that I was fooling everyone. Truth is no one cared. I created those little stories so that my brain would accept it. I fooled myself so many times. When I got in the car at work, I believed I was going straight home. When I stopped at the shop, I believed I was only going to buy 1 bar. When I walked out with 15 Cadbury's cream eggs, a Galaxy Cookie Crumble and a family size bag of onion rings, I believed that I had bought so much because it would last a week. No one was more disappointed in me than me when I arrived at my house and all of it had gone. Luckily for me, no one else knew. And everyone knows that whatever you eat in the car, it doesn't really count! Stuff the wrappers under the seat, dust yourself down and pretend it never happened.

I've buried my head in the sand and my feelings in food for so long that it was second nature. By the time covid came along I was already in the high 20s in weight and I felt powerless to stop it. Over covid, the comfort eating got worse, my movement and mobility lessened and, before I knew it, even standing for moments at a time caused me tremendous pain. I felt so trapped in my own body.

The enormity of the task ahead of me to lose all of this weight was just too much and I could not see myself being able to do it. So I didn't even try.

That is why Parkrun was so instrumental in changing my thinking. I didn't have to think about losing 20 stone, I only had to think about walking a little bit faster than the week before. And I can do that. Every week, I give it my very best. When I get a PB (personal best time) I am so proud of myself. When I don't get a PB, I know I have given it my all. Sometimes I will have a twinge or feel a bit poorly and I will allow myself the grace to be a tiny bit slower because I know in the long run, I need to keep myself injury free. I am making choices. Positive choices. Choices about what I do and how I do it. I am not depriving myself - I am actually giving myself what I need. I am feeding my soul instead of my stomach (and yes - I do know how cheesy that sounds but I am leaving it in because it is true).

I realise that I am the person that has my light. I am able to do this. I can put one step in front of the other. I believe in me. The way I view myself has changed. A few weeks ago, during a Parkrun, I passed someone who said to me 'you are strong.' For the rest of the walk, I thought about that statement and I decided that I agreed with it. I am strong. I feel in control of me and I feel worthy of making better choices. I do not eat chocolate any more and it's been a long time since I craved it. I can tell you that I do not even think about chocolate nowadays. More on this later! Sure - every now and then, I will see something and I will get a flash of need/greed. I have even given myself permission to have it to test the strategy. I truly don't want to. It no longer gives me comfort. Last night, Sophie opened a box of Maltesers whilst we were watching a film. She offered me one and I said 'no thanks' without even thinking.

Who even am I????

I am a person whose head is in the right place.

Your turn:

What about your head? Is it in the right place? Let's do a little self reflection.

Write down 5 words to describe yourself.

1. .
2. .
3. .
4. .
5. .

Now write down 5 words that a loved one or friend would use to describe you. If you find this difficult, ask someone you trust to write it for you.

1. .
2. .
3. .
4. .
5. .

Look at both lists - is there anything you would add or subtract if you had a magic wand?

_____
_____
_____
_____
_____
_____
_____
_____

Think about your **overall goal** which you set in chapter 1. If you achieve this goal, **will it add anything to or strengthen** something on your list? Write down what it will add or strengthen:

_____
_____
_____
_____
_____
_____
_____
_____
_____

Now look back at the thing you have decided to do to put your dominoes in motion. Is doing that thing adding to or strengthening something on your list? Name it.

If it is strengthening or adding to your list, how do you feel about that?

You've found a time machine - it's not a great one though - you can only go back 1 day in time! What would you tell yesterday's self to do to make today even better. Write your message..

You've found another button on your time machine which allows you to send a text message to your ten year old self. But the message has to be 20 words - no more, no less. Write your message.

Remember, you will never know what you are capable of until it is done. Just because something hasn't worked before does not mean it never will. At one point in time you could not walk or talk or …ride a bicycle. Can you imagine if we all stopped trying to walk because we fell on our bums a few times when we were 11 months old! We are all capable of greatness. Even me ….even you.

Believing that you are worth it is key and it is the bravest thing you can do. It is also the scariest.

We often don't try because we are afraid that we won't succeed and we are always our harshest critic. I know - I hear me in my head and that woman can be nasty!

See yourself as the child you once were: curious and full of potential. Talk to yourself like you would talk to that child - with kindness, compassion and encouragement. That child needs you to be the adult that loves and supports them.

Chapter 4

Eating with the enemy

I am a proud Irish woman - Dublin born and bred. Northside of Dublin and, to be exact, I am a Coolock girl through and through. What's so special about that I hear you say (maybe not - but it would be handy if you did because I'm about to tell you).

Coolock is the home of the Tayto Crisp factory (think Walkers in Britain and 'chips' everywhere else) AND the Cadburys Chocolate factory. I grew up twixt and between the salty savoury deliciousness of Tayto Cheese and Onion crisps and the sweet, creamy goodness of the Dairy milk - which, by the way, is actually good for you - after all, it has a glass and a half of milk in every bar and what's better for you than milk! Combine the 2 and you've got a cocktail of sweet savoury deliciousness. I never had a chance!

My sister, Teresa, and I (I actually have 5 sisters and 4 brothers - proper Irish Catholic family) joke that we grew up on the fumes of the Cadburys factory and it became our oxygen. Infact, at Easter time, we would relish cracking our eggs in half and using them as an oxygen mask, just breathing in the sweet, sweet air. It was a ritual. You could always tell when someone had been in the Easter eggs because they invariably had the tell tale chocolate oval giving them away. We never learned.

Living in the shadows of these confectionery giants had its pros and cons.

The pros: first of all, so many of our neighbours worked in Cadbury or Tayto. Getting in with those neighbours meant one thing: factory seconds! The Cadbury's factory had an onsite shop where they sold the chocolate that had … gone wrong I suppose. Maybe the wrappers had gone on wrongly or the conveyor belt had backed up and the bars got stuck together. That used to happen to Chomp bars a lot. A tangle of Chomps was a glorious thing to get your hands on.

Anyway, the onsite shop sold these 'seconds' in large bags to the workers. They capitalised on this and you could buy BAGS of this stuff off them for little or nothing. Everyone's ma had at least one bag hidden somewhere in the house. Our mission, and we always chose to accept it, was to find that bag. We tried to nibble away at it at a rate that she wouldn't notice - she always noticed! Sometimes, she would tell you, and only you, where the chocolate was and she would let you get a bar out for you and her to have with a cup of tea.

I felt like Charlie Bucket living between our very own Chocolate/Crisp factories and the Oompa Loompas were selling cheap knock offs at every corner. It was heaven.

So that was the pro.

The con? The exact same thing. Chocolate was everywhere. But it wasn't the ease of access. Infact, the fact that it was hidden and a little bit forbidden made it so much more enticing. Throw in a game of hide and seek to boot and you have every child's treasure island fantasy. Chocolate was a treat on special occasions and it was a reward if you were good. It was a distractor when times were hard and it was a comfort when times were tough. And it was tasty.

I can safely say that, from as early as I can remember, I was a chocoholic. I used to scoff at people who could open a bar of chocolate, have a square or two and then put it back in the cupboard! It was unthinkable. Don't get me wrong - I loved the Taytos - but I was **in love** with chocolate. It was delicious and comforting and always there - it was reliable! You could depend on chocolate to give you a lift. It was a temporary reprieve from whatever else was going on. And that sugar hit! I lived for it.

Like any drug though, the more you have, the more you need. And I was seriously addicted. Towards the end, it was not unusual for me to eat 12 Cadbury's cream eggs, a family size bag of onion rings and a few Bounties as a palate cleanser. Daily. I didn't buy bars, I bought packs. Packs of four at first …. and then boxes on the internet.

I hid it everywhere. If I wasn't eating it, I was thinking about eating it or I was planning where and when I was going to get it. I was an addict.

When I decided that enough was enough and that I had to make a change, I knew that the chocolate had to go. Whatever else I did, I knew that I could not moderate chocolate. Just as an alcoholic cannot just have 'the one drink', I know that I cannot have chocolate.

So I stopped.

Will power at first. Fear was a help - diabetes, high blood pressure, cholesterol - I didn't want a chocolate casket. But I knew that even that would not last long. I have tried - and failed - so many times before.

So this time I did something different.

Abi has just finished her A levels- she was studying psychology. She told me about systematic desensitisation which is where you gradually expose yourself to something you hate and add some nice associations. One minute, you're afraid of snakes but over time, you build up your tolerance until one day you're holding one and thinking about getting one for Christmas. It made me realise that it was possible to 'recode' your brain and I wondered if it was possible to do the opposite - to recode your brain to reject something you are addicted to. I looked into it. It is. It is called aversion therapy. This is where you associate negative things with something you want to stop doing.

I also used to be a smoker (I know - family history, morbidly obese and smoking -I was a sedentary timebomb!) and a heavy smoker at that. I like to think that when I do something, I am all in! I read Alan Carr's book, 'The Easy way to Give up Smoking', not believing for a minute that it would work. I read it to the end, smoking all the way, then gave up on the last page. Didn't smoke for years. Till I did. The brain will get you that way - you know the story 'I'll just have a puff ….it's only when I have a drink ….I only have a few a day …'. A tale as old as time. Then my daughter Abi found out. She told me that she was scared. She knew I was already at risk, being so overweight. She knew the risks of smoking (damn those effective programmes in schools) and she was worried. I got out the Alan Carr book and started at Chapter 1. I have not smoked since.

When I'd given up, someone once asked me how long I'd given up for. I said 'forever'. They explained that they meant how long had it been since I had had my last cigarette. My brain had completely misunderstood the question because I had switched my thinking. I didn't count the days or weeks since my last one because it was immaterial. I was never going to smoke again.

So I knew it was not only possible to recode the brain, I knew that I had done it before - twice!

Now before I tell you what I did, I need to give you a trigger warning here. I am going to be describing some really disgusting things. If you're queasy, take it easy. Still read it. It's important but it is foul.

Because my addiction was so ingrained in comfort eating, I had to focus on rooting out that association. So I made a list of things that disgust me. You know, the sort of stuff that makes you retch just thinking about it.

These are mine:
- Mould of any kind: I have a memory from childhood of eating a jam sandwich that tasted a bit funny. I turned over the bread and found that the underside was riddled with mould. I was still chewing on a mouthful and all of a sudden I could feel the fur in my mouth and the smell in my nostrils. I felt like it was growing in me. I vomited immediately. Since then, just the thought of mould is enough to make me gag. It has taken me 3 attempts to finish this paragraph.
- Snot 1: when I was in primary school, the boy that sat beside me always had a runny nose. I don't mean he was a bit sniffly, I mean he had a permanent river of snot that ran from his nose into his mouth at all times. Every so often, he would stick out his tongue, curl it up and just suck that stuff into his mouth. It made me want to crawl out of my skin.
- Snot 2: Fast forward many years, I am on maternity leave for Sophie and I attend a coffee morning at Abi's school. Coffee in hand, chatting

away, I see a little lad running around, living his best life. 'Bless' I thought. Till he turned around and I saw the river. I was immediately transported back to St Francis of Assisi Primary School. Then, to my horror, he runs over to the plate of biscuits. Ok. 'Breathe' I says to myself - 'he'll grab one and be off on his business'. No, he picks up each biscuit, has a sniff and then **puts it back** on the plate. Every time he lifted one to his nose I held my breath: would he hit the snot river this time? We were lucky the first 2 times. He came close but there was no contact. The third time, we had literal lift off. Contact was made, the biscuit scooped and trailed all the way back to the plate. At this point, I thought I was having a fever dream. I had no idea what was being said in the group around me - I was fixated on the plate and **that biscuit**. Then, almost in slow motion, one of the mums reached across, plucked up **that** biscuit and inhaled it - snot and all. I had to leave.

- The tongue: back in time again - childhood, summer: my Auntie Colette and Uncle Willo took me on a day out down to the country to visit a pair of old uncles who were farmers. I was a Dublin girl so I was delighted to get a chance to visit a farm. Till I got there and smelled it. 'Ok - suck it up, it smells like it smells. Deal with it,' I told my seven year old self. But it was bad. Then it was lunch time and we were all called to the table. The uncles had put on a fine spread for us. They were bachelor brothers in their 70s and they did things old school. Pot of spuds, skin on, slathered in butter. Delicious. Pot of cabbage, piping hot and also slathered in butter. Delicious. Pride of place in the middle of the table - a cow's tongue. It had been boiled to within an inch of its life. It sat there, steam rising up off it as if it were the breath from the very beast who owned it. The taste buds were glistening with droplets of juice. Uncle 1 lifted the knife and hacked a chunk off, taste buds and all, and generously plonked it on my plate. I had to eat every last bit of it.

Ok - they are my most disgusting memories. I decided to associate those memories with chocolate. I literally sat down with some chocolate and visualised them. What each scenario looked like, smelled like, felt like, sounded like, tasted like. I pictured them in as much graphic detail as I could. Then I picked up a bar with a bumpy top and I remembered that tongue sitting on the table. I ran my fingers over the top and I visualised the bumps of the taste buds. I remembered how chewy and difficult it was to swallow. I took a bite and connected the bumpy, chewy texture back to eating that tongue, with the smell of the farm in my nose. I remembered the uncle's fingernails, caked with earth, as he hacked at the meat. I heard the scrape of the knife and winced when I remembered how he had picked up a stray piece of meat, chucked it on my plate and then licked his fingers. I imagined that he had opened the bar and handed it to me, dripping with tongue juice. I visualised eating the chocolate and the tongue at the same time.

Then, I opened a pack of chocolate digestives and recalled that coffee morning - every sight, every sound, who was there, what I was wearing. I visualise that child and I merge him with Seamus from school (not his real name - actually don't know anyone called Seamus which you might think is unusual for an Irish person!) I see that river of snot. I see him stick out that little tongue and suck that snot right into his mouth. I hear it cascade. Where does all that snot come from? Why is it so stringy? I see him picking up every biscuit and bringing it to his nose. I see the snot connecting to the biscuits. I see him wipe his nose with the biscuit in his hand. He touches every single one of them. As I am imagining all of this, I am holding biscuits in my hand. The chocolate is melting and they are sticky and warm. I put some of the biscuits back inside the pack, put a piece of mouldy bread in after them and then chuck the other biscuits in on top. I smell the pack and I also smell another piece of mouldy bread.

I imagine the mould growing inside that pack of biscuits… I still have that pack. I have let them grow old and soft and god only knows what that mould is doing inside of it. They are open on the table in my office. Whenever I crave chocolate during the day, I look at that pack and I retch.

Then I picked up the last piece of chocolate I will ever eat and I put it in my mouth. I did not chew. When it hit that 'melty' stage, I visualised that river of snot and remembered the sound of hocking and that little tongue cupping and sucking. I pictured that scoop of snot and the trail that followed and made its way into that poor mother's mouth. I imagined that the chocolate in my mouth was Seamus' snot - gloopy, sticky, green, runny snot.

I could not swallow that chocolate.

This was my ritual. I have no idea if that is how you do aversion therapy - I am no expert. All I know is that it turned my stomach so badly that I could not eat the chocolate or the biscuits in front of me. Since then, I have regularly revisited my revulsions. I don't do the whole ritual. I just remember what I did and how it made me feel. At first, I actively and purposely recalled this whenever I had a craving. Then it became a daily revisit.

The car was my danger place so I did my visualisations every day when I got in the car. I don't recall all of them all the time - I pick and choose. I play with them to add a detail here and there. I like to keep them fresh! Now, whenever I crave chocolate, I immediately select one of my revulsions and it turns my stomach. I notice that I am craving less and less. Because it has been such a long time since I have eaten chocolate, I have broken the addiction to sugar and the revulsions have helped me to disconnect the substance from the feelings of comfort.

I am free.

Your turn:

Do you have an 'enemy' which you know will sabotage your success? What is it?

_____
_____
_____
_____
_____
_____
_____
_____
_____
_____

How does that thing make you feel?

Positive	Negative

What does it do to your body?

_____
_____
_____
_____
_____
_____
_____
_____
_____

How does it affect you achieving your long term goal?

_____
_____
_____
_____
_____
_____
_____
_____
_____
_____
_____

What would your life be like if you stopped this thing? Really think about this and write about it in as much detail as you can. Everytime you think you are finished, ask yourself - what else?

_____
_____
_____
_____
_____
_____
_____
_____
_____
_____
_____
_____
_____
_____
_____
_____

Are you willing to stop doing this thing?

If the answer is no, that's ok. You may well be able to control your enemy. Move to the next chapter but be mindful of letting this thing sabotage you.

If you are willing to stop the sabotage, go to the next exercise.

What are your worst revulsions? Write about these in as much disgusting detail as possible!

_____
_____
_____
_____
_____
_____
_____
_____
_____
_____

Once you have your revulsions, find a quiet space to begin the associations. If you have to look up pictures on the internet to help you to visualise, do it. If you can get something that smells, even better. Have you got a texture or something you can feel to help? Try to use all of your senses to associate the taste, smell, feel, sound and look of your most repulsive thoughts with your 'enemy'. Do this as often as you can till you can recall the disgust whenever you get a craving. If there are particular times or places that trigger you, prepare to get repulsive!

Tick the boxes that apply to you below:
- ☐ Nothing matters more than your goal.
- ☐ You can recode your brain.

Chapter 5

Graft

My first Parkrun took me 1 hour and 26 minutes. I knocked 9 minutes off my time the next week and I was on cloud 9. I've said it before and I'll say it again: the support at the Warrington Parkrun is beyond amazing. You know the angel of the Parkrun that I mentioned in my post - well, her name is Ashley. She contacted me through that FB post. Guess what she does for a living? She's a mermaid in training! You couldn't make it up.

I see the same people every week and they always make me smile. A 'nearly there' here and a 'keep going' there gives me a little lift. There are times when I am pushing it and my legs are begging me to stop when I will get a high five that will literally shoot energy through me and I will be off again.

I set myself a target in that post to get my time under 1 hour. My goodness - people really got on board with me on that. As my times began to creep down, people would congratulate me as they ran past me. They knew my times and they were willing me to get there. They were invested.

On the 5th November 2022 I got down to 1 hour, 1 minute and 4 seconds. It was tantalisingly close. The next week I finished bang on the hour - 1:00:00. It was excruciating. The following week, 19th November 2022, I finished in 59:59. You could not have written it. The marshals went wild - I cried, Darryl cried, Sophie didn't cry but she also didn't disown me for crying. It was like I'd won a marathon.

The marshals at Warrington are a special kind of special. Hail, rain or shine - they are there. Christmas eve, Christmas day, New Year's eve, New Year's day and every Saturday in between. They are walking the track at 7 o'clock to make sure it is safe for us. They stand at their points shouting encouragement and willing us on no matter the weather. They are the first to congratulate and the last to leave. I have dedicated this book to them because they have been at my side throughout this journey. It was a pivotal turn in my journey when I realised that while I **had to do it myself**, I **didn't have to**

do it by myself. They have literally walked by my side and metaphorically held my hand through it all. They are genuinely good people who are genuinely happy for others. When I get a PB now, it is like they have achieved it with me and in truth they have. As I puff and pant around the course, they will greet me with such warmth that I immediately stop regretting getting out of bed. Their shouts during those last few metres truly lifts my legs and pumps my arms to squeeze the very best out of me.

Every week I do the best I can. It became important to me to be able to do that. I started adding activities to my week to help me to get better. In the early days, I was in a lot of pain when I finished - my joints and my muscles just weren't used to it. So I started to go swimming to ease them. Now I do this about twice a week. I fit in some midweek walks wherever I can. I wanted to work on my strength and cardio but exercise was hard on my joints so I joined an aqua aerobics class. Bev, the instructor, is a walking inspiration. She has lost 11 stone and is now an aqua instructor herself. Her classes are so motivational and she really pushes you to your limit. I do 2 classes back to back every week and I love her. At the start of her class she always explains that she will show us the moves but we set our own pace - and then she reminds us that we never have to do anything we don't want to - not just in the pool - ever. The repetition of that every week has really helped it to sink in. Whatever I do, it is because I love it, not because I 'have to' do it. I've started to do yoga at 9 o'clock on a Sunday morning and I never thought I would be able to do that. It is a slow flow beginners class but Lauren, the instructor, gently encourages you to give a little bit more every week and I can feel the difference in my strength and flexibility. Lauren has helped me to balance 2 things I have never been able to hold at the same time : kindness to self and pushing myself. I have either been super strict, 'feel the pain and do it anyway' to the point I have nothing left and then I swing to 'kindness' - the wrong kind of 'kindness'. Through this class, I have learned that my body is actually capable of so much more than I thought but I should also listen to it and be kind to it when I find my edge.

My attitude to food has also totally changed. Gone are the days of food being best friend or enemy. Instead, I began to look at food as …. and this is a crazy concept so strap in….just food.

I've always known that food functions as fuel for our bodies and that it can be enjoyed for its many flavour combinations. Over my adult life, my relationship with food has swung from extreme to extreme on this spectrum. I either ate whatever I wanted, whenever I wanted it and in whatever quantity I wanted it or else I was on rations!

Depending on what plan or diet I was following (or not), I would see food in terms of points, syns, free food, red food, green food, good food, bad food, naughty or nice.

I associated food with 'treats' and celebrations. There were foods I could eat and foods I shouldn't eat. But there is nothing more tempting than forbidden fruit though is there? The more I deprived myself of something, the more I wanted it. That's why I had to do the aversion strategy - I knew I would get to a point when I would want to eat chocolate and willpower wouldn't be enough. I had to sever the comfort connection.

I then began to think about what my attitude to food overall was doing to my head. I realised that I had been telling myself a very damaging narrative for years:
- ➤ Certain foods are bad and those are the foods you want.
- ➤ If you want bad things, you must be bad.
- ➤ But don't worry; you can try to be good.
- ➤ To be good, you need to only eat the good food and avoid the bad food.

- Lots of people can do this so it should be easy.
- Except it is not. You can't do it.
- You must be very bad.

Now I am not saying that these thoughts were actually in my head – but these are definitely the messages I have been giving to myself. I was eroding my self-belief and self esteem over and over again. I was convincing myself that food had more power over me than I had over myself.

And I was the one giving it that power.

So I looked at what it actually is:
- Protein
- Carbohydrates
- Fats

It is not comfort. It is not love. It is not powerful.

I felt like Dorothy in Emerald City and I'd just found the 'wizard' behind the curtain. There is no yellow brick road, there are no ruby slippers – there is only you – and science! And this is the best bit of the science: Your body burns a set amount of calories just by living – this is called your Basal Metabolic Rate (BMR). If you move more, your body uses more calories. If you eat more calories than you need, you will gain weight. If you eat less calories than you need, you will lose weight. You can control this.

What's more, I realised that all those plans I had followed in the past are really just the exact same science disguised in all sorts of smoke and mirrors. They were all just hiding the fact that if you used up more than you consumed, you would have a net loss. There is no mystery. It is science but it is not rocket science!

Of course it is more nuanced than this but this is the basic tenet. I know what you are thinking – you are thinking that I must be out of my brain to think that this is a revelation. **EVERYONE** knows this. True. Full disclosure - I've known it for a long time. It is not news.

What is new is that now I **ACCEPT** it.

I have spent my life trying to shortcut the science. This plan or that plan would be the key. Drink this and don't eat that and you too can be skinny. Get beach ready in 2 weeks: short cuts, quick fixes, easy to follow and all too easy to fall off.

I had to accept that I needed to change and it would be hard work. I was able to offset the difficulty of what I had to do by focusing on why I was doing it and remembering how important it was to me. I drew confidence from the SCIENTIFIC FACT that when your calorie intake is less than your output, your body will burn off excess fat. I drew strength from the FACT that I could control both of those factors.

There was no big secret.

Burning fat was just a matter of knowing the facts!

Your Turn:

You are going to review your calorie input and output. Review the last 7 days – it has to be real. You can work out your calories by looking at the nutritional information on food and you will easily find lists of calories burned on the internet.

However, I found that the best way to do this is to download an app. There are loads to choose from and you don't have to pay big money for them; in fact, lots are free. For example, I use FatSecret – input your age, weight etc and it works out how many calories a day you should consume. You can also add exercise - type and duration - and it will work out how much you've used. Eat more to gain weight. Eat less to lose weight. I don't know if this is the best app - it is the one that I found first and so I'm sticking with it.

I have listed a few apps below for you to explore:
- FatSecret - free or pay for premium
- Myfitnesspal - free or pay for premium
- Controlmyweight - free or pay for premium
- Loseit! - free or pay for premium
- NHS weight loss plan - free
- Mynetdiary - not free
- Noom - - not free

Once you start looking, you'll be overwhelmed by the choice. Don't let it put you off. My advice - choose one of the free ones, as long as it can count your calories and your exercise, you're good to go.

Job 1: Don't make any changes. Don't try to 'be good'. Record what you eat and what you do from an exercise point of view. Use the grid below to record your totals.

	Calories in	Calories to live + exercise	+/-
Day 1			
Day 2			
Day 3			
Day 4			
Day 5			
Day 6			
Day 7			

How did you do? Over the course of 7 days are you in calorie deficit or calorie surplus? Record by how much below:

Another bit of science here – and this is very rough science so bear with – 3,500 calories is about 1lb in weight or 0.5 of a kilo.

- ☐ So, over those 7 days, if you have used about 3,500 more than you have taken in, you will most likely have a loss of 1lb / 0.5 kg.
- ☐ If, over those 7 days, you have used less than you have taken in, you will most likely have a gain.
- ☐ If you've more or less used the same as you've used, you will have maintained.

Tick which one applies to you.

Are you happy with your tick?   Yes or No

If you are not happy with your tick, look back at your food and activity logs of the past 7 days. Is there anything on there that you could change? This could be a change to your weekly activities or it could be a change to what you eat.

Identify what you **could** change and write it down here:

Go back to your overall goal from chapter 1.

Big Question: Is achieving that goal worth making some changes?

Yes or No

Explain why below:

Are you **going to** commit to making a change? Yes or no

If so, go back to your list of things you could change and select the ones you are willing to do.

Are you **able to** commit to tracking your calorie intake and output daily?   Yes or no

What do you need to do to make the change(s)? Make a list

_____
_____
_____
_____
_____
_____
_____
_____
_____
_____
_____
_____
_____

This is you taking control. Fair play!

Chapter 6

If only it really was that simple

My life is SO different now to how I was living a year ago. A year ago, when I couldn't stand without pain. When just walking around my block caused my heart rate to rocket and I had to take rest breaks. A year ago when I couldn't walk up my own stairs. A year ago when I was wearing size 36 clothes. A year ago when I spent my weekends hiding from the world, in bed, because my working week took too much from me and I hadn't got a shred left to give my family.

But don't get me wrong here: yes, I have lost a chunk of weight - I know people who weigh less than what I've lost so far -but I have a long way to go to get to what is a 'healthy' weight. I am still morbidly obese - I am not out of the health woods yet! The difference is that I feel healthier now. I live healthily now. I don't have to wait to lose another 8 stone to feel like I've accomplished something. Everyday is an accomplishment. That's why I am writing this now. I don't have to wait till my BMI is in an 'acceptable' range to share the transformation I am having. I can share it now because I am living my success now and you can too.

Having said that, every day isn't a picnic. I have hard days and I have very hard days. Old habits can be hard to break and they are sneaky little things that try to sneak back in when you're not looking. They hide themselves in traditions and the familiar. Mince pies at Christmas, Easter eggs at Easter and a chinese/indian/chippie 'treat' on a Friday!

The thing is to not let them sneak up and ambush you! Everything is ok and everything is allowed as long as you plan for it. When I know I have an event coming up, I am a little bit more careful the week before. I don't feel bad when I've been out - I know I made a choice, I enjoyed it and I'm still in control. I am looking at the big picture and know that I need to be able to live like this and that includes special occasions. I will use my calorie calculations to work out what I am willing to accept this week. I might work out that going to that wedding is going to put me in surplus for that week. That is ok. It will be a small gain and by the following week or the week after, it will be gone. As long as I am mindful, I don't mind.

All of that is fine.

But what happens when you are doing everything 'right', when you are doing all that you can, when you are not having a treat or a night out? When you are tracking your calories and you are in deficit? What about when you are doing all that and the scales aren't moving or your time goal isn't getting any closer? What happens then?

In the past, it was at this point when I would falter. 'The plan' had stopped working. There was no point continuing. I was stupid to think it would have worked in the first place. That only works for other people who aren't as big/bad/lazy (insert any negative adjective here - I've been through them all) as me. This is not for you. This is not what you really want. What you really want is chocolate. You deserve it….

And then I jump off that wagon with the same sort of gusto that I jumped on it with. I dive into self-loathing and swim in despair. There is a special kind of twisted joy in proving your unspoken fear right - you were never going to actually make it anyway.

I have hit that phase over the past 11 months and I know that I will meet it again. It is part of the cycle. My first 4 stone came off easy peasy (ish). Over the last 11 months I've had 2 kinds of plateaus - either my weight wasn't shifting or my Parkrun time wasn't improving. Both of those things are important to me and I've had to battle through some very long plateaus. It has really tested my resolve.

After Christmas, I hit a period of time when my weight just would not shift. I was doing everything 'right' but I just couldn't regulate my weight loss . I'd lose one and put on 2, lose 3 put on 1 …. Up and down for weeks! I put on about half a stone / 7 lbs / 3kg. In the past when this has happened, I have lost belief in the long term goal to lose weight. This time was different. I made it different.

I keep coming back to my overall goal: to be fit and healthy in body and mind. I go back to how I measure success in this goal. I ask myself if the numbers on the scales are my only measure of success. They are not.

Then I ask myself if the numbers on the scales are amongst the most important measures of success I have identified - they are not. Being able to live my life with my family, being able to move, feeling healthy, feeling happy are all measures that are much higher on the list.

I ask myself if the numbers on the scales were even a reliable measure of success. They are not. I could be losing weight by not eating healthily or starving myself. The number on the scales might go down but all of those other, more important measures would suffer.

I ask myself if I am willing to jeopardise all of those other measures of success, all of the very real benefits that I feel every day because of a number. I am not willing to do that.

My scales now give me markers in time to track my journey. They help me to reflect on what I am doing and what my body is doing. They sometimes nudge me to amend my activities or review what I am eating. They are not how I measure success.

I am purposely writing this using the present tense because I am very much still in the thick of this journey. I have called this chapter 'If only it were that simple!' because I know that 'Graft' is not always enough. Breaking those old habits is tough.

Sometimes , I will find myself falling into old rabbit holes. 2 of my big triggers are letting the scales dictate success and becoming overwhelmed by the size of the task. I have almost eliminated the first trigger. Focusing on how I measure success has really helped me to do that. Infact, focusing on the measures of success helps with the second one too. The measures are not final and finite. They are incremental. When the literal and metaphorical weight of the task ahead of me becomes too much, I focus on the now. What have I achieved today? I allow myself to feel the smallest of victories. I don't look at what has to be done, instead I look at what I have achieved and I allow myself to feel proud. I then ground myself in the reality that if I have done 'that', then I can also do 'this'. This is evidentially and factually true. Having multiple measures of success means that I can always draw on at least one to pull me back from the brink.

This is how I have stopped sabotaging myself. This is the difference between then and now. In the past, when I have reached a plateau I have allowed my head to distract me. I have allowed my head to think illogically and cruelly and I have not allowed myself to see the full measure of my successes. I have not allowed myself to feel my successes at all. I was saving up my happiness for the day when I would be a size x and weighed x.

It was too hard and too distant. No wonder I fell into the comfort food trap so often.

No more.

Your turn:

Have you sabotaged yourself in the past? I know the answer will be yes - we have all done it! Think about the last time this happened.

When and where did it happen? Who was there? Write down everything that you can remember about it.

What did you do exactly?

How did you feel, physically in your body, when you sabotaged yourself?

How did you feel emotionally when you sabotaged yourself?

What were you thinking when it was happening?

What were you thinking afterwards?

___

What are your sabotage triggers? They are sneaky so think hard to identify and name them - that way they can't sneak up on you!

___

Think back to those goals and the measures of success you have set for yourself. Think back to how important these are to you. In fact, write them down again right here to ensure that they are front and centre in your mind. Add some if you would like to.

How can you sabotage the sabotage?! What are you going to do next time this happens?

Remember, one of the biggest sabotage tricks is for your brain to tell you that you've messed up and ruined it all. Your brain will try to tell you that one slip has undone everything.

Let me ask you something - if you were putting £10 in a bank every week for 6 weeks and then one week, you couldn't - would you abandon the account? Let the bank keep the money?

What if it's worse than that? One week you have to take out £40. Would you abandon the account then?

Or would you recognise that you are still in credit, you still have a bank account and next week is a new opportunity to bank a tenner!

I'd put money on you keeping that bank account!

Chapter 7

Running up that hill

The other plateau I have reached over this year is in my 5K finish times. For the first 6 months, my PBs were coming in thick and fast. I was knocking big numbers off my time and I could feel myself getting stronger and stronger every week. It was exhilarating.

After I broke the 1 hour barrier on the 19th November 2022, my next goal was to get below 55 minutes. I was driven.

I began to look at what I was eating in terms of what is best for my body. I wasn't following any particular diet or plan - I was just being mindful about what I ate and how many calories I was consuming. The only 'rule' I had was that I aimed to have a daily deficit. Thinking about food in terms of protein, carbohydrates and fats helped me to make choices about what I wanted to eat. I began to play with what I was eating and not just how many calories I was taking in. I noticed I was much more sluggish when I ate more carbs and I didn't like the feeling. On the flip side, I noticed that I felt much better when I had more protein.

I was discovering all this after 19th November and, lo and behold, I was knocking chunks off my Parkrun times. I was giving it my all every week. I was doing 2 aqua classes a week, I was swimming twice a week and I'd just started yoga. I felt fitter than ever. I had the odd twinge in my hip when I walked but the days of being in constant pain were gone. My mood was better and my head was in a great place. Even when I hit that weight loss plateau, I worked my way through it. I didn't panic..

I hit my next goal of breaking 55 minutes on the 11th February. 5K in 54 minutes and 41 seconds to be exact! Before I go on, I just want to share that there is nothing that tastes as good as achieving a target. It is just brilliant - the adrenaline is pumping and it feels like anything is possible. Once I caught my breath and was able to stand up straight, I was delighted!

Of course, I immediately set my sights on my next target: a 50 minute 5K. It took me from the 20th August to 19th November to get under the hour. Then it took from 19th

November to 11th February to get under 55 minutes. By my reckoning, I figured I should be smashing the 50 minute mark by mid May. Easy.

Nope.

I suppose it was inevitable that there would come a time when I couldn't walk any faster. I hit that wall in March 2023. I was giving it my all every week. But I just could not shave any time off. I got down to 54.04 on the 11th March but after that I hit wall after wall after wall.

But I had learned during the weight loss plateau that it helped to go back to focus on my measures of success to help me stay grounded and focused. I rationalised that even though my time was not getting better, my head and my body was. I could feel the difference. I was still enjoying the Parkrun and I was more active than I had been for years. I would not sabotage myself.

Now back in Dec 2022, there was a buzz among the Warrington parkrunners. One of our regulars, Jean (a wonderful woman in the veteran women's age 85 -90 category) had just got a PB of 47 mins 46 seconds. I was still riding the wave of getting my time under an hour and I had got a PB the same week of 59 mins 32 secs. I had gone all out to do that so when I heard about Jean's

PB, I was in awe! I vowed to watch out for her in future weeks to see how she did it.

Try as I might though - I just couldn't spot her. She was too fast! Then on the 17th June, months into my finish time plateau, I was lucky enough to find myself walking behind the elusive woman herself. I hadn't been able to better my time since March so I was excited to spot her because I happen to know that if you want to get better, you have to look to the best. When I saw Jean, I vowed to keep up with her. So I followed - or at least I tried!

I saw how she swung her arms and powered through in a steady walk. She was mighty. When it came to the down slopes, she picked up her feet and ran. 'Snap' I thought- I'd been doing that myself for a little while so I was delighted to have the same strategy. It was actually the trick that helped me to get under the 55 minute mark. Well done me!

I carried on following/stalking Jean. Then came an upward slope and I felt sorry for her...and myself. The Warrington route is a fairly flat one but there are a few slopes that have been my nemesis since day dot. The muddy slope to the field has nearly finished me a few times! I was excited to see how she tackled them. You could have knocked me down with a featherlight feather when I saw her strategy- she only went and **ran** up them. I couldn't believe my eyes.

I resolved then and there that I would do the same.

So, as I approached the same slope, I told my brain to run. Nope - legs wouldn't listen.. Next slope - up runs the legend. I ordered my brain to run and what do you know: run I did - for about 5 seconds.

I really tried to keep up with Jean that day but I could not. She finished in 51 mins and 20 secs. I finished in 54 mins 05 secs. I couldn't keep up… but I did get the best time I'd had in a long time. I was so happy and deeply inspired. Since that day, I've been working on the legend's strategy and what do you know? I only went and got myself a PB of 53 mins 07 secs within a couple of weeks. It is not the legend's time nor is it sub 50… but it's a lot closer.

Jean didn't just gift me with a Parkrun strategy, she also gifted me with another shift in my mindset. I don't want to beat the legend's time - I want to be her. And I don't mean when I am her age. I mean right now. She logged her first parkrun in 2021 and has well over 80 under her belt. Look at her times and you will see that she is not out for a stroll out there. She is going for it. She is some woman for one woman.

I had been so pleased with myself when I started running down the dips at Parkrun. 'Look at me -I'm running!' Proud as punch. But I would have **never** considered running up the slopes had I not seen the legend herself do it. The strength of her body to be able to break into those runs and the strength of her mind to just dig in and do it. And that was the mind shift for me - don't fear the hard bits.

The hard bits are where the wins are. Jean knows this. Jean owns the hard bits.

I had a think - I realised that I had become complacent. I had stopped pushing myself. I pretended I was. Just like I used to pretend that I wasn't going to buy a shed load of chocolate and scoff it all in my car in the 30 minutes it took me to get home.

Now this is the important bit. Somewhere in my brain, I knew that embracing the hard bits is the key to succeeding. I knew it when I registered for Parkrun and turned up the next day even though I was terrified. I knew it when I turned up week after week when it was killing me just to stand, never mind walk. I even knew it when I wrote that Facebook post and admitted I had eaten myself to 30 stone. I knew it. But I allowed myself to forget it.

So I need to Worzel Gummidge this and get my SMART head on. I know it helps me when I set myself a **s**pecific and **m**easurable goal. My current hard bit is getting my Parkrun time under 50 minutes - as a goal, that is specific and measurable. I also know that I respond best when I believe that my goal is **a**chievable and **r**ealistic. Getting under 50 minutes is definitely doable - literally hundreds do it every week at Warrington. And that's just one of the hundreds of Parkruns across the world. I had built it up in my head as something really difficult. It is not. Lastly, I know I need a **t**imeframe for this so that it becomes real. I have done 44 Parkruns so far. If my new milestone was to get under 50 minutes before I hit my 50th Parkrun, this would be smart, measurable, achievable, realistic and timebound. SMART. That's what I'm going for next.

And that is Jean's gift to me. You have to keep owning the hard bits - forever. You are in it for the long run. You don't have to kill it every week. You have to be SMART about it - plan, pace and work it. And just when you think you have cracked it, you go back to the plan and you ask yourself - what next!

Your turn:

Is there something that you have been avoiding doing/starting because it seems too difficult? Set yourself a goal to conquer this - make sure it it SMART - specific, measurable, achievable, realistic and timebound:

_____
_____
_____
_____
_____
_____
_____
_____

Visualise you have achieved this difficult thing. Describe how you are feeling - in detail:

_____
_____
_____
_____
_____
_____
_____
_____
_____
_____
_____
_____

Describe what is happening in your body

Describe what you think about yourself, having achieved this.

Describe who else is there. What are they saying/doing?

_____
_____
_____
_____
_____
_____
_____
_____

Visualise the time and place when you have achieved this 'impossible' thing? See yourself there - use the exercises you've just done to step into how you are feeling, what is happening in your body, what you're thinking, who is with you, what they are saying/doing. Now take **one step back *in time*** from this achievement. What did you do **directly** before this point in time in order to achieve it?

Write it down:

_____
_____
_____
_____
_____
_____
_____

Now take one step back from this point. What did you do **directly before this point in time** in order to get here? Write it down:

Now take one step back from this point. What did you do **directly before this point in time in order to get here**? Write it down:

Keep stepping it back, till you reach yourself in the present day. Don't rush it - step it back, one step at a time.

Look back over your steps. You've just written an action plan to achieve something that you once thought too difficult.

Now put that plan in motion.

Chapter 8

Food for thought

When I hit my weight loss plateau back in January, I focused on my measures of success and it helped me to stay on target. But it was hard. Those old demons are strong and they get stronger when they see you at your most vulnerable.

At that time, I was being so disciplined. I was logging my calories, increasing my activity and it just didn't make sense that I wasn't losing. I was staying on track but I could feel myself wobbling. I knew that my aqua instructor, Bev, had lost 11 stone so I decided to hang back after class one evening to talk to her. I am so glad I did.

She gets it. Been there, done that and worked hard to get those tiny tank tops. She's had those same dark nights of the soul. She began by asking me the basics:

- Was I drinking enough water? Yes

- Was I sleeping enough? Not really but I would work on it
- Was I being active? Yes
- Are you varying your diet? Yes
- Was I eating enough? What?

I thought she had misunderstood me somehow and she could see that I was confused. She went on to explain that if I wasn't eating enough, then my body would overcompensate and slow down my metabolic processes. She explained that when she went through her weightloss journey, she never let herself go hungry. Even now, she can happily eat a whole chicken for dinner!

Yet another mike drop moment.

I went home and reviewed my food diaries on my app. I was not eating enough. I had let the fear flip me back to old thinking - eating = bad; not eating = good and I had been gradually reducing what I was eating so that, over time, I had started to deprive myself again. It happened incrementally so I didn't notice it but that is the beauty of keeping a log. It's all there for you to review.

I looked back - week after week - and I saw it happening. I think I panicked that I had overindulged over Christmas and I slipped back into my old ways. As a matter of fact, I actually didn't over indulge at all - yes, there were days I went over but most other days I went under so it all balanced out. I don't know why I let my head get to me - all I know is that I did.

So I began to eat more - I thought about the amount of protein I was eating, the amount of carbs and the amount of fats. I increased the amount of protein I was eating in particular. All of a sudden, my weight started to move down again. It was slow but it was consistent.

And when I hit a similar bump in April, I went back to look at my logs again. I saw that I had fallen into a different kind of rut this time - I was relying on the same meals and snacks week in, week out. I remember Bev asking me if I was varying what I ate and that wasn't a problem at the time. Now I saw that my food was very samey. I mixed things up and, lo and behold, the numbers on the scales began dropping again.

I began to look at food as more than the comfort that it used to be and the fuel that I had come to see it as. I thought if varying my diet had had such an impact, what else could I do? My eldest sister Jacinta has always waxed lyrical about the virtues of nuts and seeds. I decided to look into it and what do you know - she was only right. (I will never live that sentence down!) I discovered the benefits of nuts like almonds, brazils, cashews and walnuts -they are high in protein and fibre and they contain nutrients like vitamin E, potassium and magnesium. I'd always heard that nuts have a very high fat content so I had stayed away from them. This is true, they do, but if you have them in moderation they are so good for you. They boost your immune system, your metabolism and some experts even say they are good for your cardiovascular health.

Seeds are another tremendous source of goodness -linseeds, sunflower seeds, pumpkin seeds, chia seeds, flax seeds. They are all full of fibre, vitamins and minerals and they are great for a healthy diet, especially if you eat them raw and unsalted. Again, you have to be careful with these as they are also high in fats but it is the 'good' kind and the omega three fatty acids in them actually help to speed up your body's fat burning metabolism.

I was in a research hole at this stage and I was getting excited. If Jacinta was right about the nuts and the seeds, was she right about the dates, prunes, dried apricots and raisins? Yes she was. What about drinking your own urine? Only joking - she never recommended that but I think if she had, I would probably do it at this stage because she was right about the rest.

I bought the lot and made up my own 'trail mix'. I have a couple of spoonfuls in the morning with 150g of greek yoghurt. It is a high calorie breakfast but the boost to my weight loss has been ridiculous and within weeks I noticed that my hair, nails and skin were also much better.

This was such an important lesson for me - living healthily is not just about the foods you don't eat - in fact it has very little to do with that. It is about the foods that we choose to eat. The point of this chapter is not for everyone to go out and start collecting nuts and to eat like squirrels - although they are spritely little chaps. The point is that I started to think about **what** I was putting in my body, not just how much. It is about being mindful and selective.

It is not about starving yourself - it is about feeding yourself well.

Your turn:

Let's do a checklist to review how you are doing?:

- ☐ Are you still focused on your overall goal?
- ☐ Are you remembering your measures of success?
- ☐ Is your head in a good place?
- ☐ Are you managing your 'enemy'?
- ☐ Are you tackling the hard things?
- ☐ If you are trying to lose weight, are you creating about a 3,500 calorie deficit over the week?
- ☐ If you are trying to maintain, are you balancing your calorie intake with your output?
- ☐ Are you drinking enough water? The NHS says you should drink between 1.5 and 2.5 litres per day.
- ☐ Are you varying your diet and eating smart? Nuts, seeds, berries etc -you may have your own recommendations from your own sisters/friends! Do your research though
- ☐ Are you sleeping enough?
- ☐ Are you active?
- ☐ Are you eating enough? Especially protein?
- ☐ Are you drinking your urine? No? Good. Don't do that.

If you've ticked all of these - great. Crack on.

If you've not ticked some of them, what can you do to get your tick? Write down what you are going to do. Don't just think it - write it down:

_____
_____
_____
_____
_____
_____
_____
_____
_____
_____
_____
_____
_____
_____
_____
_____
_____
_____
_____

Keep this list handy - remember how the mind likes to play with us. We all need to check in with our checklist to stay on track.

Chapter 9

Run, Nic, Run!

Jean's strategy gave me a wake up call. I thought I was pushing it as hard as I could. I was even starting to feel a little bit sorry for myself - the negative thinking hadn't quite snuck back in but it was definitely prowling around! Once I had my SMART goal, I began to think about taking my next step - could I run?

At the time this thought was dropping, I was 23 stone 8lbs. This was still extremely overweight and I was very scared of doing myself an injury by doing something that was too high impact on my body. Running for very short spurts up and down little slopes is very different to running for 40 minutes which is the high end of average for Parkrun. I can't do that.

So I listed the activities I was doing weekly:

- ☐ Parkrun 5 K weekly
- ☐ 2 aqua classes per week
- ☐ 2 swimming sessions per week
- ☐ 1 yoga class per week
- ☐ Midweek walk

Well aren't I doing everything I can, I thought self-righteously to myself.

Was I?

That list is what I had been doing. I went to my logs and looked properly. I had to admit I was not being as consistent as I had been. My midweek walks had turned into mid month walks and I had started to skip one of my weekly swims. I had started to slip.

I keep coming back to how the mind is tricky. You can fully believe you are doing everything 'right' - until you make yourself sit down and have a think.

I suppose it makes sense though. I mean I got to the size I was because I was an expert at deluding myself. I was eating this because I was hungry. I was eating that because I deserved a treat. I was only going to have one…box. I didn't just have a quarter pounder meal and a wrap from the drive through on the way home and then come in and eat my dinner. Not me. I cannot understand how I am so big!

Being honest with myself has been the hardest part of this journey. What's even more difficult is that I have to keep forcing myself to do it. I've learned that when I think I've cracked it, I probably need to have a proper think just to check I'm not pulling the wool over my own eyes.

You see - just there - right in that paragraph, I've not been honest. Because being honest is actually not the hardest part of the journey. The honest to goodness most difficult thing about this is being kind to myself when I've not been honest. Being kind to myself when I've had a slip. Being kind to myself when I don't get something quite 'right'.

I find that so hard. I beat myself up over the smallest of things and I jump on myself so quickly - I even did it in the previous paragraphs. I also have a tendency to obsess over something. That can be a good thing - remember the nut/seed/fruit research - I was in that hole for a while! But I learned a lot and I now eat much more mindfully than I did before. It can also be a bad thing - same obsession: 'why didn't I listen to Jacinta? why haven't I looked into this before? how do I not know this?.....' Beat, beat, beat. My self-talk is actually so much worse than what I just wrote but there's such a thing as too much honesty!

I've examined this tendency to beat myself up to get to the root of it. I know I like to do things well, so that's a part of it. I like achieving things - who doesn't? It might be a childhood full of A Team shenanigans but I absolutely love it when a plan comes together so I get very disappointed when things don't work out. Level 1 thinking there. Need to go deeper.

Down to level 2 - do I get upset when other people don't get something quite 'right'? Not at all. Quite the opposite. I am the last person to jump on someone if something hasn't worked. I am very conscious of not beating others up. In fact, I know that failing is very much part of the learning process and I welcome it. 'Show me someone that never fails and I'll show you someone that is not trying' and all that! I am the sort of person who will help someone else to get back up, dust themselves off, ask them the most annoying question which is 'what have you learned from it?' and then encourage them to go again.

So why don't I do that for myself?

Down to level 3 thinking here - you have to sit at this level for a bit and really root around. Why don't I offer myself the same sort of compassion I give to others?

Maybe I am not kind to myself because beating myself up starts a cycle which has been my go to my whole life. Lets just think this through:

- I don't get something quite 'right'
- I beat myself up
- I feel stupid/unworthy/incapable …..
- I now feel horrible
- I need to feel better
- How can I feel better?
- I can eat …
- That was nice. I feel better now. But…..
- I shouldn't have eaten that!
- AWWW! Now I've done something not quite 'right' again
- I beat myself up

You get where I am going with this. The cycle is vicious and relentless. Why do I allow this cycle to continue?

Level 4 - it's getting dark here. Do I do this on purpose? Maybe. You know when you're in a bad mood so you pick a fight with your partner/some other poor innocent. You don't know why you're in a bad mood but you know it's there and you need to let it out so you pick at some scab or other. If the recipient is feeling particularly brave, they might even say to you - 'what's wrong with you - you're spoiling for a fight'. Of course, you'll deny it down to the ground but deep down inside, you know it is true. Am I doing this to myself on purpose? Not the making mistakes bit - that's human. I mean, am I picking a fight with myself? Do I do that on purpose? Do I do it because I know it will lead to me self comforting through food and, therefore, I know that it will actually lead to me feeling better, even if it is only for a very short period of time. What if by being mean to myself and not giving myself any 'rewards', I purposely fall back on old habits to get some kind of reward?

Big thought here: what if I allow myself to feel good about my achievements instead of ignoring them? What if I were to make myself feel better by being kind to myself and telling me it's ok when something doesn't quite work out? What if I just offer myself the same compassion I give to others? Then I won't need to do the whole self comforting through food thing at all!

Level 5 thinking - flood lights on this level! This is why it has never worked for me before. On all of those other plans and programmes, it is shameful to struggle. The programme is good. You are the problem… you are letting yourself down, you are letting the programme down and you are letting everyone else who believes in it down.

The cycle is so transparent to me now:

- You start well - the 'plan' is great, you are great.
- You fall off - boo: the 'plan' is still great, you are the bad person. Get back on.
- You get back on - hooray: The plan is great, you are a good person again. Stay on.
- You are on plan - which is great by the way, but it is a struggle. The pressure not to fail is huge.
- What's that, you've fallen again? Boo? You really are bad at this aren't you?

There is no grace, no kindness. There is doing it right and doing it wrong. There is no credit for just doing it.

Level 6 thinking - never been here before. Doing it is all that matters. There will be highs and there will be lows. You will get it right and you will get it wrong. You will plateau and you will shake it up. You will remember your goals and know that the bigger picture is worth it. You are worth it. You will measure success in lots of different ways and you will give yourself credit for the smallest of victories. You will be honest with yourself and you will be kind when you fail. Because you will fail but you know that from every failure, there is the opportunity for deeper learning and deeper understanding. You will do all of this and you will keep doing it because you know that you are not alone in this.

We all feel the pain. Just keep going.

Just keep doing it.

Your turn:

What do you do when you don't get it quite 'right'?

How do you act?

How do you feel?

What do you think about yourself?

What do you do when others don't get it quite 'right'?

How do you act towards them?

How do you feel about them?

_____
_____
_____
_____
_____
_____
_____

What do you think about them?

_____
_____
_____
_____
_____
_____
_____

Are you kinder to yourself or others?

_____
_____
_____
_____
_____

What are the signs that you are being unkind to yourself?

What can you do to stop that cycle? Name a concrete thing which you can do to pull you back from unkindness towards yourself.

Chapter 10

Doing it!

Since I had my level 6 epiphany, I have been actively noticing my self talk and challenging myself when I am being unkind or have negative thoughts. Sometimes they are easy to catch and other times they can be quite tricky. For example, have a look at this thought process from a paragraph in chapter 9:

At the time this thought was dropping, I was 23 stone 8lbs. This was still extremely overweight and I was very scared of doing myself an injury by doing something that was too high impact on my body. Running for very short spurts up and down little slopes is very different to running for 40 minutes which is the high end of average for Parkrun. I can't do that.

I broke down these thoughts and really examined them. I discovered that this was a blocking thought: Let me show you:

- *At the time this thought was dropping, I was 23 stone 8lbs.* This is a fact. No issue here

- *This was still extremely overweight.* This is also a fact. No issue here.

- *I was very scared of doing myself an injury by doing something that was too high impact on my body.* This was an emotion that I was feeling. It is a real fear and sometimes fear is a good thing. It stops you from doing something dangerous. Is this fear valid in this case? Yes. If I did too much, got injured and couldn't stay active, I know it would really mess with my head and there would be a danger I would spiral. I was right to have caution.

- *Running for very short spurts up and down little slopes is very different to running for 40 minutes which is the high end of average for Parkrun.* This is also factually very true. No issues here.

- *I can't do that.* This is the blocking thought.

Ok - I found the thought. It was hiding in amongst some strong facts. If I hadn't caught it, I would have just accepted the status quo: 'I can't run'.

But I did catch it and I flipped it. What **can** you do then?

- I could commit to doing my midweek walk again- and if I can run down dips and up slopes for short bursts in Parkrun, then I can do that midweek too. I can punctuate the walk with little bursts. They don't have to be fast. The movement of running is different to walking, so just doing this for 30…60…90 seconds would make a difference. I can set my own targets and set my own pace and it wouldn't have a severe impact on my joints.

What else could you do?

- I could get my bike out and go cycling - cycling is low impact on the joints and is really good for your cardio health and building stamina.

What else could you do?

- I could start swimming twice a week again.

So I had 3 options right off the bat. I could have kept going and thought of some more but I find that you don't actually need loads of ideas in life, you just need to **do** one.

I thought about which one would bring me the most joy. I decided that I hadn't been on my bike for a long, long time and I actually used to really love going out on bike rides. The weather was really nice - in fact, it was great cycling weather. What's more, Sophie had got a bike for Christmas and she hadn't had much of an opportunity to use it. I would love to go out with her on our bikes. I asked her if she was up for it and, Sophie being Sophie, she was.

Now we go out on bike rides. Sophie leads the way, plotting out weird and wonderful routes around the local area. I put my complete trust in her to get us out there and back. I have to - I have no sense of direction whatsoever. Darryl and I also hop on the bikes and have little spins out together, stopping off somewhere scenic for a cup of coffee. They've become like little dates for us. Sorry - yes I wrote that. But I'm leaving it in because it is honest.

Once I felt comfortable with the bike rides, I then reintroduced the midweek walk but it was a midweek walk with a bit of spice! Calm down - I just mean I do spurts of running every 5 minutes or so. It is very slow, it is very low impact but it is helping me to find my running style and building my confidence. I now know that I can run - I just can't run continuously for 40 minutes - yet!

I fit in the extra swims when I can. If I can't, I don't beat myself up. I have tried out a beginners pilates class - I didn't like it as much as yoga but I will give it another chance before I make up my mind.

The increase in my activities is helping with my weight loss but more importantly, I am feeling fitter than ever. I ran up the stairs the other day to get something - I literally ran. I noticed it ¾ of the way up (because I was knackered) and I couldn't believe it.

I am still keeping my food and activity logs and I am mindful about what I eat. My mantra is that as long as I am mindful, I don't mind. I know that whatever goes in can be worked off and I have to live in the process. This is doing it - forever.

I regularly use my checklist to make sure that I am on track. I keep my goals and success measures updated - the overall goal to be fit and healthy in body and mind has not changed but I add SMART mini goals regularly so that I am always working towards something and I have lots of opportunities to celebrate. I think about the level of importance something holds for me and I make mindful choices. This helps me to see straight when I start to lose the plot!

I make sure that I am honest with myself.

When I check in with my head and I reflect on my self talk, I use Bernard Meltzer's advice:

Before you speak, ask yourself if what you are going to say is true, is kind, is necessary, is helpful. If the answer is no, maybe what you are about to say should be left unsaid.

However, I do it slightly differently - I ask if what I'm saying to myself is true, is kind, is necessary, is helpful?

If the answer is yes, then I take action. Sometimes I have to give myself hard messages but as long as they are true, kind, necessary and helpful then I know that I have to listen.

If the answer is no, then I ask myself why?

Why am I saying something to myself which is untrue?

Why am I saying something to myself which is unkind?

Why am I saying something to myself which is unnecessary?

Why am I saying something to myself which is unhelpful?

I know that talking to myself like that will not help me to be fit and well in body and mind. So I work out what is going on in my head to cause me to do that. I then work on that thing.

I need to do this so that I don't slip into sabotaging

myself - this exercise also helps me to stay honest with myself.

And in the interest of being honest, let's just put this out there: there is nothing in this book that you didn't know already. There is nothing in this book that I didn't know before I started my journey. But knowing and doing are two very different things.

It is my hope that reading my story and completing each 'Your Turn' section has helped you to step onto your own path of doing it.

The next 'Your turn' section is just for you. Use it to record your thoughts, your small victories, your sneaky blockers masquerading as facts. Rework your measures of success. Write a nice note to yourself every now and then. Write to yourself as if writing to a friend you love deeply. I will be doing exactly the same in mine. This means that we can carry on doing it together, that none of us are alone and that all is possible.

Nic x

PS: If you're ready to start doing it and you want to come on your journey with me, join DOING IT 2 online. You can sign up at nicdowardcoaching.com or by scanning the QR code.

Your turn:

ABOUT THE AUTHOR

Nic Doward is a 46 year old wife and mother. She has been married to Darryl for 19 Years and they have 2 daughters. They live in Warrington in the north west of England.

Nic was born in Dublin, Ireland, and is the youngest of 10 children. She moved to England in 1999 for love (Darryl) and stayed for…love again (also Darryl).

She is the headteacher of a secondary school and is a professional coach with experience in leadership, performance and transformational coaching.

Nic knows that she is blessed every day to have such a wonderful family, a wonderful job and a wonderful life.

Nic finds it weird that she has written all that about herself, using 3rd person narrative!

Printed in Great Britain
by Amazon